Great Dreams

David Adams

Contents

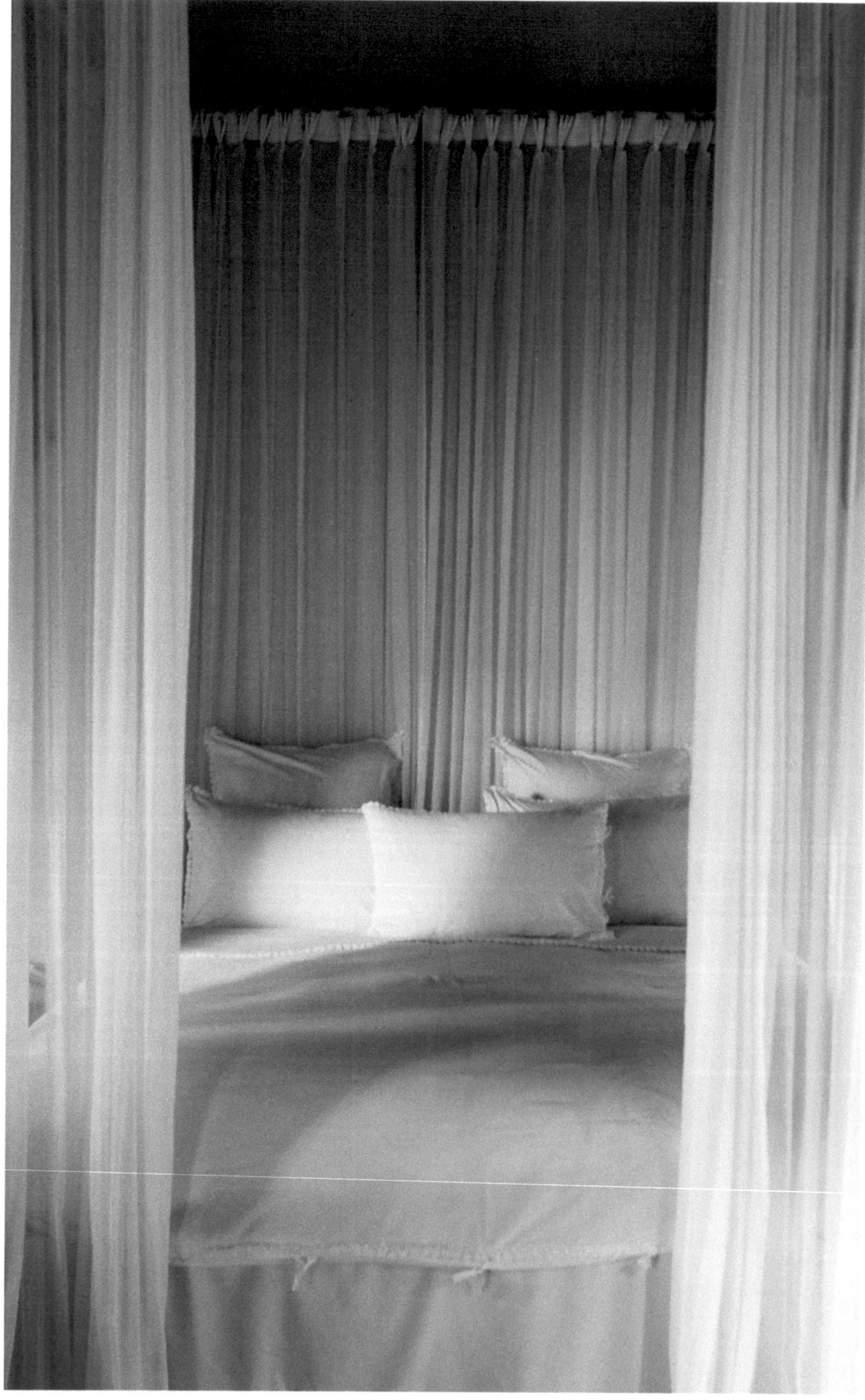

Introduction

Every night, you need an average of 7–8 hours of sleep. Sleep is as essential as air, water, or food. Now, ponder this: How much have you invested in enhancing the comfort of your bedroom in the last five years? Could it be that you're resting on an uncomfortable mattress and an old pillow handed down from your parents?

Let's momentarily step away from the quest for a cozy bedroom because that alone won't guarantee a good night's sleep. In this book, you'll discover a plethora of simple and effective lifestyle and sleep hygiene recommendations that can enhance your sleep quality and quantity.

Even if you've already optimized your bedroom comfort and maintain a healthy lifestyle, persistent poor sleep might indicate an underlying sleep disorder. There are over 70 known sleep disorders.

The recent coronavirus pandemic has cast a shadow over various aspects of our lives, significantly impacting sleep patterns.

And then there's stress – the ubiquitous culprit behind many sleep disorders.

The bed is our whole life, here we are born, here we love and here we die.
Guy de Maupassant.

Creating a Clean Bedroom

In almost half of the cases, poor bedroom hygiene is the primary cause of sleep disturbances among city dwellers. Disruptions may arise from an uncomfortable mattress or pillow, a restless "neighbor" on a narrow bed, or noise infiltrating from the street or the adjacent wall.

Much like our daytime attire, our bed plays a crucial role in our nightly comfort.

Hygiene mandates the same consideration for a bed as it does for clothing: it must be convenient and comfortable for the sleeper. The bed should not impede the evaporation of moisture from the skin's surface or hinder the proper dilation of skin vessels, ensuring normal body warmth and efficient removal of excess heat from the skin.

Our comfortable bed

Choosing the Right Bed for Quality Sleep.

The width of the bed is paramount, particularly when accommodating two people in a double bed. Optimal comfort may be compromised when people sacrifice it for additional space and resort to sleeping on sofas. However, sofas often lack comfortable mattresses and prove highly uncomfortable for sleeping. Fortunately, manufacturers have introduced folding anatomical sofas with fully-fledged mattresses, saving space during the day while ensuring a comfortable sleep experience at night.

For an ideal choice, consider beds made of natural solid wood. Beds upholstered in natural or artificial leather (eco-leather) are also hygienic. Eco-leather, created by applying a microporous polyurethane film onto a fabric base, is a highly breathable material. In terms of properties, eco-leather closely resembles natural leather and is safe for use.

Here's a practical tip: smell the material of your prospective bed. Ideally, it should not emit a strong odor. If you detect an unpleasant chemical smell, it's advisable to explore products from a different manufacturer.

Choosing the Right Mattress for Quality Sleep

The world of mattresses boasts an overwhelming array of options, sometimes leaving even the sellers themselves bewildered by the diversity. Individual preferences in mattress firmness also vary widely; some prefer a soft mattress while others opt for a firmer one. Material choices, like wool, may be ideal for some but trigger allergies in others. While specific mattress recommendations can be challenging due to these diverse needs, adhering to certain general principles is advisable.

Given that mattresses cannot be checked from the inside, reliance on the manufacturer's reputation and personal usage experience becomes crucial. Invest in a mattress from a reputable manufacturer, as serious companies prioritize their reputation and offer products with a well-maintained price-quality ratio. Generally, the more expensive the mattress, the more technologically advanced, reliable, and environmentally friendly it is.

To extend a mattress's lifespan, consider using protective covers made from natural materials with a waterproof membrane layer, shielding the mattress from dirt.

Anatomical mattresses are often deemed more comfortable and beneficial. Designed to maintain the correct body position and spine alignment during sleep, they distribute the load evenly by conforming to the body's contours, alleviating individual areas of excess pressure.

The common question arises: what distinguishes anatomical from orthopedic mattresses? The answer is straightforward: there's practically no difference.

When making a mattress selection, it's advisable to lie on it for 10-15 minutes in various positions – back, side, and stomach – directly in the store. This provides ample opportunity to assess comfort and predict individual preferences. The key is to feel no particular pressure points or tension in your body.

If you discover that the mattress's firmness doesn't meet your expectations during use, adjustments are possible. Special thin mattresses or toppers, also known as comfort correctors, allow you to fine-tune the mattress's hardness.

For those allergic to animal hair, opt for a mattress without wool or horsehair content. Consider products treated with anti-allergenic compounds or featuring rubberized cotton upholstery.

The Ideal Pillow for Sweet Dreams

When selecting pillows, prioritize those with environmentally friendly natural or synthetic fillings, discouraging the growth of dust mites. Options like natural latex, polyurethane foam, and holofiber are recommended.

For those drawn to down or feather pillows, opt for high-quality products crafted through meticulous manufacturing processes, including sorting, repeated washing, superheated steam drying, degreasing, antiseptic impregnation, and special anti-allergenic and antistatic treatment.

Ensure that expensive down pillows come with certificates confirming the purity of raw materials and correct processing for both usability and safety.

Regardless of the filling, pillows should undergo regular cleaning or be washed at least once every six months, if the manufacturer permits. Consider replacing any pillow every three years for optimal hygiene.

If waking up with a headache or discomfort in muscles or the cervico-thoracic spine is a common occurrence with a regular pillow, consider trying an anatomical/orthopedic memory foam pillow. Typically made from elastic material, these pillows have a rectangular shape with a depression for the head in the center and raised areas along the edges. The anatomical shape promotes a parallel head position to the body, relaxing the neck and shoulder muscles.

It's worth noting that an adjustment period might be necessary for orthopedic pillows. Initially, they may seem less comfortable and soft compared to regular ones. However, after a few nights, the disappearance of headaches and muscle tension in the neck becomes apparent.

Once you've determined the type of pillow and filling, lie on it for 10-15 minutes in the store, both on your back and on your side. Your personal comfort during this trial is the primary criterion for selection.

Choose a pillow on a mattress with the same firmness as your home mattress or the one you plan to purchase. If you sleep on your side on a hard mattress, a thicker pillow is needed to ensure your head is parallel to your body. On a soft mattress, a thinner pillow is sufficient for optimal head positioning. Hence, the pillow and mattress must complement each other.

In larger stores, the pillow selection area often includes three mattresses: hard, medium, and soft. Test the pillow on the mattress that feels most comfortable for you.

The Perfect Blanket for Cozy Nights

Blankets play a crucial role in ensuring a comfortable sleep environment, and they can be categorized into winter, summer, and all-season varieties. A well-selected blanket should maintain an ideal temperature, neither too hot nor too cold, providing the necessary thermal conductivity and air circulation.

Here's a brief overview of common types of blankets:

Cotton Blankets:

Pros: Affordable.
Cons: Noticeable weight, tends to absorb odors, less practical.
Wool Blankets:

Pros: Ideal for those who prefer warmth, excellent heat retention, good moisture absorption, beneficial for various health conditions.
Cons: May be too warm for some, relatively heavier.
Bamboo Blankets:

Pros: Lightweight, breathable, environmentally friendly.
Cons: Limited warmth, may not be suitable for very cold climates.
Down Blankets (Duck or Goose):

Pros: Light, resilient, durable, excellent heat retention, good air circulation.

Cons: More expensive, not suitable for those with allergies to down.
Synthetic Blankets (Sintepon, Holofiber, Polyester Fibers):

Pros: Light, durable, hypoallergenic, machine-washable.
Cons: Limited moisture absorption.
Choosing Based on Preference:

For Warmth: Wool or down blankets are suitable, providing excellent heat retention.
For Slight Coolness: Thin blankets with synthetic filling are ideal, offering a lightweight and breathable option.
Considerations:

Health Conditions: Wool blankets are recommended for musculoskeletal and cardiovascular issues, diabetes, and excessive night sweats.
Allergies: Opt for hypoallergenic options like synthetic blankets if allergies are a concern.
Washability: Synthetic blankets are convenient for machine washing.
Ultimately, the perfect blanket choice depends on personal preferences, health considerations, and the desired sleep environment.

Creating the Ideal Sleep Environment: Bed Sheets and Bedroom Atmosphere

Getting a good night's sleep involves more than just a comfortable mattress and pillows. The environment you sleep in, including your bed sheets and bedroom atmosphere, can significantly impact the quality of your sleep. Here's a guide to optimizing your sleep environment:

Choosing the Right Bed Sheets:

Material Matters: Bed linen can be made from various materials such as cambric, cotton, linen, satin, or silk. Choose a material that feels pleasant to your touch. Experiment with different types to find your preferred choice.

Quality Check: If the bed linen color transfers to your skin or fades excessively after washing, it indicates low-quality dye. Opt for high-quality materials and dyes to ensure safety.

Breathability: The fabric should allow normal air circulation and temperature regulation. Whether you prefer sleeping without clothes or in pajamas, choose sheets that enhance your comfort.
Optimizing Bedroom Atmosphere:

Temperature Control: Experiment with room temperature to find what suits you best. While some studies suggest better sleep in a cooler room, individual preferences may vary. Aim for 20-22 degrees Celsius.

Dust-Free Zone: Remove dust-collecting items such as carpets, tapestries, and decorations to maintain clean air. Regularly wet clean and ventilate the bedroom.

Lighting Considerations: Use chandeliers and lamps with warm-colored light before bedtime to minimize melatonin suppression. Ensure darkness during sleep, and consider a night light for convenience.

Morning Light Exposure: In the morning, provide more light to aid waking up quickly. Open curtains to let in natural light, especially in the darker seasons. Light alarms can mimic sunrise in the mornings. Ensuring a Quiet and Relaxing Environment:

Soundproofing: Make your bedroom quieter with soundproofing materials and triple-chamber double-glazed windows. Earplugs, white noise generators, or natural sounds like sea surf can aid in noise reduction.

Dark and Quiet Mornings: Ensure a dark room for better melatonin production during sleep. Use curtains and light alarms to manage light exposure, promoting a peaceful waking experience.

Creating an optimal sleep environment involves personal preferences and experimentation. Pay attention to the details, from the sheets you choose to the overall atmosphere of your bedroom, to enhance your sleep quality.

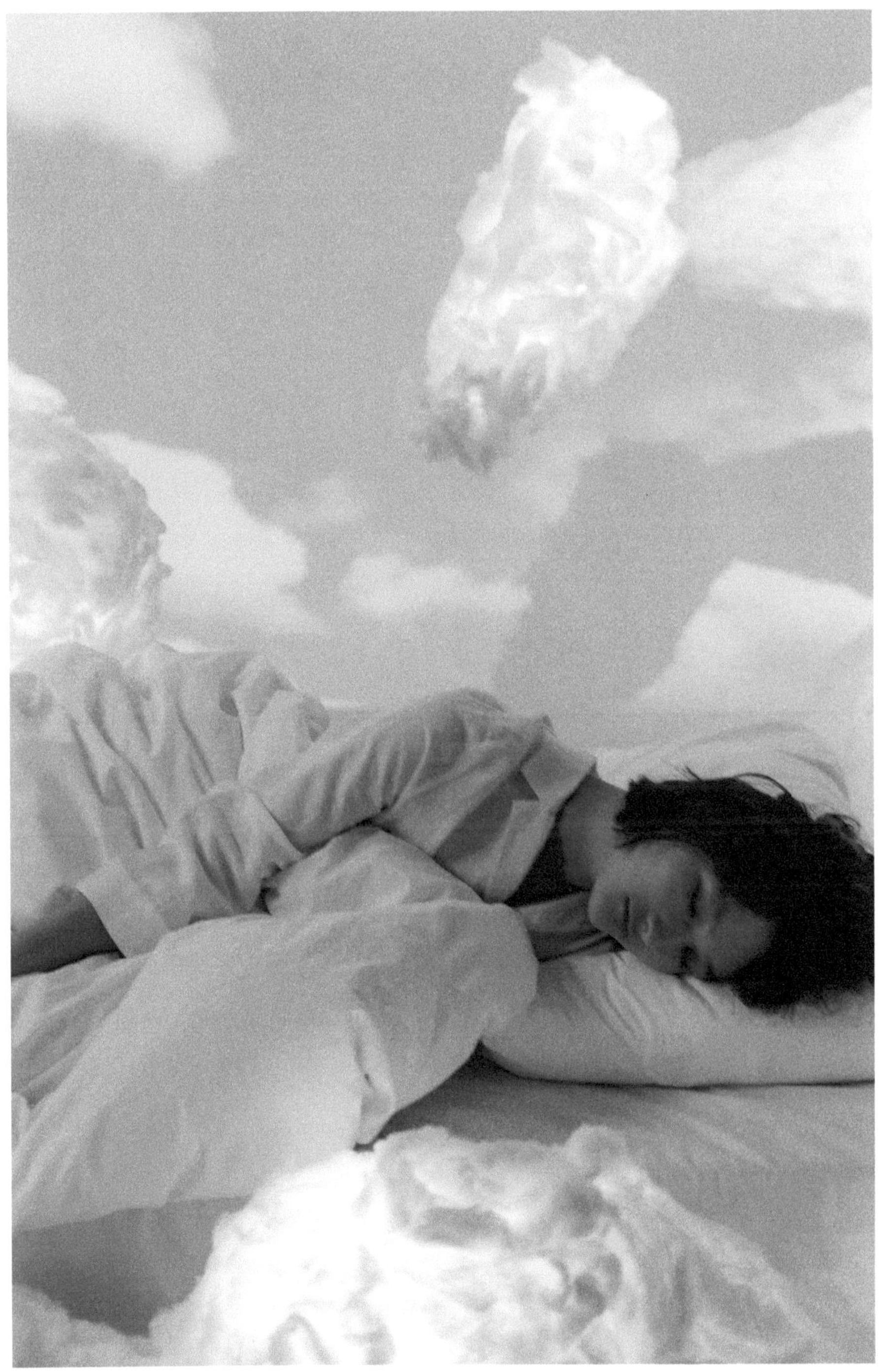

Understanding the Dynamics of Sleep: A Complex and Individual Process

The phenomenon of sleep is far more intricate than a mere state of rest or passivity. Contrary to the common perception of sleep as a downtime for the entire organism, it involves an intricate interplay of various factors, particularly within the brain. Here are key insights into the complexity and activity of the sleep process:

Memory and Brain Activity:

Active Restoration: Sleep serves as a dynamic mechanism for restoring strength and initiating a kind of "reboot" for the body.
Brain Engagement: Despite the appearance of stillness, the brain actively works during sleep. In fact, certain periods exhibit higher brain activity compared to waking hours.

Sleep Cycles and Stages:

Cyclic Patterns: Sleep unfolds in cycles, typically ranging from 4 to 6 cycles per night. Each cycle spans 1.5-2 hours and encompasses distinct stages.
Sequential Stages: The four sequential stages within each sleep cycle include:
Stage 1 (Sleep): Initial transition into sleep.
Stage 2: Characterized by K-complexes and "sleep spindles."
Stage 3 (Delta Sleep): Essential for energy accumulation and hormone production.
REM Stage: Rapid Eye Movement stage associated with dreaming and memory processing.
Unraveling Sleep Functions:

Enigmatic Second Stage: The exact function of the second stage remains a subject of uncertainty and ongoing research.

Delta Sleep Benefits: Energy accumulation and the synthesis of various hormones, such as growth hormone and testosterone, occur during delta sleep.

REM Dreaming: The brain engages in information processing, decision-making for the future, and the formation of long-term memory during REM sleep.

Individualized Nature of Sleep:

Complex Individuality: Sleep is not a one-size-fits-all process; it varies among individuals based on factors such as age, health, and lifestyle. Unique Sleep Patterns: The composition and duration of each sleep stage can differ, making the sleep experience highly individualized.

In essence, sleep emerges as an active and multifaceted process, contributing to the overall well-being of the individual. As scientific exploration continues, the intricate dynamics of sleep promise ongoing revelations about its vital role in maintaining physical and mental health.

Navigating the Mosaic of Sleep: The Dynamic Landscape of Individual Needs

The duration of optimal sleep is a personal and ever-changing aspect of human well-being, shaped by a myriad of factors. Here's a closer look at the nuanced realm of sleep:

Individualized Norms:

Genetic Diversity: Genetically, everyone harbors a distinct baseline for required sleep, spanning a spectrum from 4 to 12 hours.
Common Ground: For the majority, a well-functioning state is achieved with 7-9 hours of nightly sleep.

Life's Evolutionary Influence:
Early Stages: Newborns engage in 17-18 hours of daily sleep in segmented intervals, while preschoolers thrive with 9-10 hours at night and a brief daytime nap.

Adolescence Onwards: As children progress into adolescence, daytime naps become less essential, and stable long-term sleep patterns typically endure after 18 years.
Understanding Sleep in Older Age:

Quality vs. Quantity: Contrary to assumptions, older individuals might not sleep less; instead, sleep quality may diminish with more nocturnal awakenings.
External and Physiological Influences:

Dynamic Response: External factors, including pregnancy, increased workload, educational demands, and sunlight exposure, dynamically influence sleep needs.

Adaptability: Recognizing the evolving impact of external factors aids in adapting sleep routines accordingly.
Chronotypes: Unveiling Night Owls and Larks:

Divergent Preferences: The existence of "night owls" favoring later sleep schedules and "larks" thriving in early mornings highlights individual chronotypes.

Tailoring Sleep Schedules: Acknowledging and accommodating these preferences contributes to a more personalized and harmonious sleep routine.

In essence, the query of how much one should sleep lacks a universal response. Instead, it unfolds as a multifaceted and individualized narrative, influenced by genetic predispositions, life stages, external stimuli, and unique preferences. Embracing this diversity becomes paramount in fostering a holistic understanding of sleep, ultimately promoting well-being through tailored sleep practices.

Harmonizing the Sleep Symphony:
The Rhythmic Dance of Consistency

To orchestrate a serene night's rest, establishing and adhering to a consistent sleep schedule emerges as a cornerstone. Here's a closer look at the significance of maintaining a synchronized sleep routine:

Pillars of Consistency:

Wake-Up Ritual: Endeavor to rise at the same time every day, bridging weekdays and weekends. This practice anchors the body's internal clock and fosters a rhythmic sleep-wake cycle.
Weekend Flexibility:

Balanced Variance: While minor adjustments on weekends are permissible, extending sleep by a maximum of 1-2 hours beyond the regular wake-up time maintains a delicate equilibrium without disrupting circadian rhythms.
Cautious Approach: Prolonged sleep during weekends risks perturbing the body's natural biorhythms, potentially triggering circadian disturbances and contributing to insomnia.
Avoiding Prolonged Wakefulness in Bed:

Strategic Bedtime: Limiting time spent in bed to match the required 7-8 hours of nightly sleep is pivotal. Excessive time spent in bed may inadvertently elongate sleep duration, disrupting established routines and fostering conditions conducive to insomnia.

Circadian Harmony:

Aligning with Natural Cycles: Acknowledging and respecting the body's circadian rhythm bolsters the effectiveness of the sleep routine. This entails synchronizing sleep patterns with the natural ebb and flow of the day.
Holistic Sleep Hygiene:

Comprehensive Approach: Beyond schedule adherence, integrating other sleep hygiene practices, such as a calming pre-sleep routine and optimizing the sleep environment, enhances the overall quality of sleep.
In essence, the quest for restful nights intertwines with the cadence of consistency.

A steadfast commitment to regular wake-up times, cautious adjustments during weekends, and strategic time allocation in bed cultivates an environment conducive to sound sleep.

By embracing the symphony of consistent sleep, individuals set the stage for a harmonious and revitalizing night's rest.

Cultivating Tranquil Evenings:
The Art of Bedtime Rituals

Our lives are adorned with everyday rituals that weave seamlessly into our existence—a rhythmic dance of habits that often go unnoticed. From morning rituals like the familiar brush of teeth to the automatic retrieval of keys upon nearing home, these routines streamline our daily lives. Much like these, sleep can be cultivated into a habit, or more precisely, the arrival of the coveted drowsiness at the opportune moment. Enter the bedtime ritual—a tailored practice designed to usher in the serene embrace of sleep.

Crafting the Ritual:
Incorporate activities geared towards both mental and physical relaxation into your nightly routine. Consider a warm bath to alleviate physical tension, engage in self-hypnosis exercises, or indulge in the soothing melodies of calm music. Within the framework of this ritual, repetition of specific actions in a consistent sequence is not only allowed but encouraged.

Sequence and Repetition:
Take, for instance, the creation of a bedtime ritual. Picture this: every evening in the hour preceding bedtime, immerse yourself in the pages of a good book. Follow it with a comforting cup of herbal tea, indulge in a leisurely bath, and cap it off with a relaxation exercise. This repetitive sequence, when practiced consistently, transforms into a soothing bedtime habit.

The Transition to Habit:
Repetition is the key—engage in your bedtime ritual night after night
until it seamlessly integrates into your routine, becoming a second nature. As the ritual becomes a steadfast habit, the arrival of drowsiness
will harmoniously align with the desired bedtime.

In the symphony of daily life, the bedtime ritual emerges as a com-
posed melody—a deliberate practice that guides you into the realm of
tranquil sleep.
 Through thoughtful actions and consistent repetition, transform bedtime into a ritualistic dance that gracefully invites the gentle embrace
of rest.

Harmony of Movement: Unveiling the Power of Physical Activity for Restful Sleep

Embarking on the quest for a night of serene slumber, one often
underestimates the profound influence of physical activity—a potent
elixir for stress relief and a natural inducer of drowsiness. Harness the
inherent connection between physical exertion and quality sleep to
cultivate a restful night.

Aerobic Symphony for Sleep:
Among the myriad forms of exercise, aerobic activities emerge as the
virtuosos of sleep preparation. Engage in activities such as jogging, cy-
cling, swimming, or brisk walking to orchestrate a harmonious blend
of physical effort and tranquility. The great outdoors, with its expan-
sive canvas, amplifies the effectiveness of these activities.

Temporal Rhythms:
Timing, akin to a well-tuned melody, plays a crucial role. The optimal window for physical activity lies between 5 to 8 in the evening—a period where the body seamlessly aligns with the rhythms of exertion and relaxation. However, heed the conductor's advice: conclude your physical endeavors at least 90 minutes before the curtains fall on the day.

Balancing Act:
In the grand ballet of physical exertion, strike a harmonious balance. Aim for an optimal duration of intense activity, ranging from 150 to 300 minutes per week—a delightful dance spanning 20 to 40 minutes each day. This rhythmic cadence ensures a well-rounded symphony, blending various activities while adapting their durations to compose a melodic routine.

In the choreography of sleep, physical activity takes center stage—an artful interplay of motion and rest. Allow the grace of aerobic exercises to guide you towards the tranquil shores of slumber, creating a masterpiece that unfolds nightly, casting aside the stresses of the day.

Culinary: Nourishing Sleep Through Thoughtful Eating

In the gastronomic symphony of life, where each note influences our well-being, the culinary choices we make can significantly impact the quality of our sleep. While there isn't a bespoke sleep diet, adhering to some fundamental principles can pave the way for a restful night.

Dinner's Prelude:
Embark on the evening's culinary journey with a mindful approach. Avoid retiring to the realm of dreams on a full stomach by abstaining from indulging in a meal less than 2-3 hours before bedtime. The nocturnal menu should gracefully sidestep gaseous protagonists—nuts, legumes, or raw vegetables—to prevent any unwarranted disturbances.

Banqueting in Moderation:
Striking a harmonious balance is the key—neither should hunger be your lullaby, nor the pangs of an overstuffed stomach disrupt your nocturnal serenity. If hunger comes knocking before bedtime, opt for a light repast, perhaps a banana or an apple, to appease the nocturnal cravings.

The Caffeine Sonata:
As the day's curtain descends, it's prudent to taper off the intake of dietary stimulants, particularly caffeine. This invigorating substance, omnipresent in coffee, tea, tonic beverages, and chocolate, wields a lingering influence. Beware that certain green tea varieties harbor even more caffeine than their black counterparts.

Timing the Culinary Crescendo:
The zenith of caffeine's stimulating effects unfolds 1-2 hours post-consumption, casting a shadow that lingers for 6-8 hours. To foster a seamless transition from wakefulness to the realm of dreams, bid farewell to caffeine-laden delights at least 6-8 hours before the anticipated rendezvous with the sandman.

In the culinary ballet of sleep, orchestrating a mindful menu and timing the culinary crescendo can be transformative. Let your dietary choices be the gentle lullaby that ushers you into the arms of peaceful slumber, allowing the night to unfold in perfect gastronomic harmony.

A Symphony of Choices:
Harmonizing Sleep with Health

In the orchestral composition of a restful night, the choices we make regarding smoking and alcohol play a pivotal role. Consider these nocturnal maestros, nicotine and alcohol, and their impact on the harmonious symphony of sleep.

Nicotine's Crescendo:
Smoke less or bid adieu to the smoking serenade altogether. The nicotine in cigarettes, a stimulant more potent than caffeine, can disrupt the tranquility of your sleep. Consider refraining from indulging in this nocturnal performance at least 2 hours before you embark on your journey to the land of dreams. The curtain of sleep rises gracefully when nicotine takes a bow.

The Intoxicating Waltz:
In the grand ballroom of sleep, dance with moderation when it comes to alcoholic libations. Sipping small doses—perhaps 50 g of vodka or 200 g of wine—occasionally dons the hat of a soothing melody for a healthy adult. Yet, be wary, for in the crescendo of indulgence (150-200 g of vodka), the deep stages of sleep may find themselves silenced, replaced by a dissonant tune of interrupted and unrefreshing rest.

A Tale of Warnings:
Behold the inscriptions on cigarettes—"smoking is harmful to your health"—and on bottles of spirits—"excessive alcohol consumption is harmful to your health." These are not mere whispers; they are cautionary tales, reminding us that indulgence in these nocturnal indulgences can cast shadows upon our well-being.

In the nocturnal symphony, where each note resonates with health, let your choices be a harmonious cadence that lulls you into the embrace of restful slumber. For in the nocturnal ballet, the dance of health intertwines with every note, creating a melody that echoes through the night.

Navigating the Technological Twilight:
Charting a Course for Better Sleep

In the symphony of the night, the glow emanating from our gadgets orchestrates a delicate dance with our sleep. Let's explore the intricate notes of this nocturnal ballet and unravel the influence of technology on our journey into the realm of dreams.

A Spectrum Sonata:

The luminescence from computer screens, tablets, and smartphones, particularly in the blue spectrum, mirrors the characteristics of daylight. This spectral serenade, akin to the sun's embrace, triggers the retina to respond similarly, hampering the production of melatonin—the sleep hormone. To curate a smoother transition into the embrace of slumber, consider bidding adieu to gadgets 1-2 hours before bedtime.

A Digital Nocturne:

For those who find solace in the glow of screens even before sleep, navigate the digital dusk with finesse. Dim the brightness and summon a special filter that banishes the disruptive blue spectrum, casting the screen in hues of twilight (affectionately termed "night mode") at least 2 hours before your rendezvous with the Sandman. Modern operating systems, such as Android and iOS, graciously extend the option to automate this celestial transition, allowing your device to gracefully don its nocturnal attire.

In this technological nocturne, where each pixel paints a brushstroke on the canvas of sleep, let your choices wield the baton of balance. As the curtains of the digital stage draw close to the night, usher in the twilight hues to guide your passage into the realm of restful repose.

SLEEP DISORDERS

In the sanctuary of your carefully curated sleep haven, where the ambiance whispers tranquility, if elusive slumber still evades your grasp, you may find yourself entangled in the enigmatic embrace of sleep disorders. Modern medicine, akin to an alchemist's trove, unravels a tapestry of over 60 sleep maladies, clandestine culprits that not only disrupt the sanctity of sleep but also cast a shadow on the tapestry of life itself.

In this nocturnal odyssey, where each disorder narrates its own tale of turmoil, let's cast our gaze upon the most prevalent protagonists: snoring, obstructive sleep apnea syndrome, circadian sleep disorders, restless leg syndrome, and the elusive specter known as insomnia.

Snoring: The Nightly Serenade:
A nocturnal symphony often accompanied by unwitting duets from sleep partners, snoring takes center stage. While seemingly harmless, its persistent presence may be a precursor to more ominous sleep disruptions.

Obstructive Sleep Apnea Syndrome: A Breathless Ballet:
In the realm of dreams, a breathless ballet unfolds. Obstructive sleep apnea syndrome, a clandestine performer, orchestrates a silent struggle for breath, heightening the risk of cardiovascular afflictions and casting shadows on the tranquility of slumber.

Circadian Sleep Disorders: Time's Unyielding Grip:
Time, a relentless arbiter, may play capricious tricks on the internal clock. Circadian sleep disorders, disrupting the harmonious dance between sunlight and slumber, unfurl their disquieting narratives.

Restless Leg Syndrome: The Limb's Lament:
A nocturnal lament, the restless leg syndrome, unveils its presence
with an inexplicable urge to move, fragmenting the serenity of repose and leaving the sleeper ensnared in a tangle of restless limbs.

Insomnia: The Elusive Specter:
In the shadows of sleep, where dreams and wakefulness entwine,
insomnia emerges as the elusive specter. A fickle companion, it
eludes the grasp of rest, leaving its mark on both the night and the
waking world.

A Wakeful Vigil: Seeking Solace:
If you find yourself ensnared in the clutches of insomnia or wres-
tling with sleep's elusive companions, discerning when to extend
a self-helping hand and when to seek the guidance of a vigilant
healer becomes paramount.

In this nocturnal tapestry, where each thread whispers a unique
tale, may your journey through the realm of rest be guided by the
wisdom to discern when to tread alone and when to seek solace in
the embrace of a caring guardian of sleep.

Snore: The Subtle Harbinger of Silence Disturbed

In the symphony of night, where dreams entwine with the hushed whispers of slumber, the resonance of snores emerges as a common nocturnal companion. Approximately 30% of the adult populace engages in this nightly performance, an auditory tapestry woven with subtle complexities.

Yet, behind the seemingly innocuous melody of snoring lies a more profound narrative—a prelude or, in many cases, a central manifestation of a grave ailment known as obstructive sleep apnea syndrome, where the cadence of breath is intermittently disrupted during the sanctuary of sleep.

Insomnia's Myriad Masks: Decoding the Dreamless Realm

Within the nocturnal tapestry, where dreams weave an intricate dance, insomnia takes center stage, donning myriad masks with over a hundred different guises. It is not merely the absence of sleep but a complex interplay of factors that orchestrates this elusive companion.

To unravel the enigma of insomnia and guide restless souls back to the realms of restful repose, the pivotal first step lies in the sanctum of a somnologist—a vigilant guardian of sleep disorders. Here, the journey towards healing commences, as consultations and examinations converge to illuminate the intricate pathways leading to the restoration of wholesome sleep.

In this nocturnal odyssey, may the resonance of snores and the perplexing dance of insomnia find solace in the compassionate care of those versed in the language of dreams and the delicate threads that weave the tapestry of a restful night.

Chronicles of Restless Nights: Unveiling Coronasomnia's Silent Grip

In the shadows cast by the global pandemic's upheaval, a silent epidemic unfurls its tendrils—Coronasomnia. As the world grapples with the repercussions of COVID-19, a surge in insomnia cases emerges as an unforeseen aftermath.

The chronicles of this silent malady reveal a profound impact on sleep patterns worldwide. Express Scripts, in April 2020, sounded the alarm with unsettling data: a staggering 14.8% rise in prescriptions for sleep medications compared to the previous year. The restless nights, amplified by the pandemic's resonance, become a pervasive phenomenon, etching its presence across the globe.

Post-COVID, the specter of chronic sleep disorders looms over 20% of individuals. While speculation exists about the virus directly affecting the brain and sleep centers, scientific validation remains elusive.

The nocturnal symphony, disrupted by the virus, extends its influence beyond the infected. Stress, a common accomplice of insomnia, emerges as the primary culprit. The nervous system, under the weight of unprecedented stimuli, succumbs to hyperexcitation, denying the brain the respite of restful slumber.

Healthy sleep, a devotee of stability and routine, finds itself entangled in the chaos wrought by the pandemic. Remote work alters schedules, transforming bedtime rituals into erratic dances. Benjamin Franklin's timeless wisdom—"Weariness is the best pillow"—is forgotten as physical activity dwindles during the era of self-isolation.

In the labyrinth of sleep disrupted by the pandemic's fallout, Coronasomnia's silent grip persists. Yet, amidst the shadows, the quest for restful nights endures, seeking solace in stability, routine, and the resilience of the human spirit.

Sailing the Turbulent Seas of Stress: Unraveling Its Impact on Sleep and Life

In the tapestry of human emotions, stress often lurks in the shadows, underestimated and overlooked. Beyond mere unpleasant emotions and a few nights of unrest, stress conceals a more formidable adversary. In a staggering 90% of cases, the genesis of long-term insomnia finds its roots intertwined with the tendrils of stress.

This seemingly intangible force exerts a tangible toll on life expectancy, rivaling the impact of physical inactivity, smoking, and poor diet combined. Stress, a silent catalyst, propels the aging process forward and nurtures the seeds of detrimental habits, contributing to life's brevity. The risk of cardiovascular demise amplifies by fivefold under the influence of stress.

Yet, the response to stress is as diverse as the human tapestry itself. The magnitude of its impact, its resonance in sleep's realm, and the subsequent consequences hinge on the intricate interplay of health and psyche.

Understanding stress requires a holistic exploration—scrutinizing its triggers, predisposing factors, individual responses, and the potential for complications. For those entangled in the chronic dance with stress, a profound medical approach emerges as the beacon of hope.

Navigating the labyrinth of stress-induced insomnia demands a concerted effort to soothe the beleaguered nervous system. Practical steps unfold as a roadmap:

Eliminate Stimulants: Spare the already taut nerves from additional provocations.

Embrace Physical Activity: Fortify your defense with the antidote of movement.

Moderate News Consumption: Constrain exposure to distressing news, allocating no more than 15 minutes a day.

Establish Sleep Patterns: Maintain consistency in sleep-wake cycles, even if nighttime rest eludes you.

Avoid Daytime Naps: Delay the embrace of sleep until the nightfall to enhance the quality of rest.

Minimize Discussion of Stressors: Shelve discussions about stressors, preventing the exacerbation of internal turmoil.

Should these self-guided measures prove insufficient, the beacon beckons: seek the expertise of a specialist. As the turbulent seas of stress churn, the voyage towards peaceful shores often requires the guiding hand of those skilled in navigating the complex currents of the human psyche.